D1044554

Why Not Us?

Sandra M. & Octavian M. Braxton

Contents

All rights reserved.

ISBN:
ISBN-13: 978-1518742354
ISBN-10: 1518742351

You met me deep in my despair to show me You
would never leave me there.

You claimed because I was made for so much more.
I am Your child and I'm worth fighting for.

Though heavy with the weight of my mistakes,
You carried me and refused to let me sink under the pressure. You
meant for me to soar. I am Your child
and I'm worth fighting for.

Eyes haven't seen.
Ears haven't heard all You have planned
for me and nothing can separate me from
Your love when there's so much
more still worth fighting for.

Now I'm moving by faith and not by
sight towards victory by the power of Your might.
You're straightening out my past and opening
every door. I am Your child and I'm worth fighting for. – Brian
Courtney Wilson

This book is dedicated to anyone going through infertility and feeling alone.
You are NOT alone! You can get through this. There is light and life on
the other side.

ACKNOWLEDGMENTS

There are many people that have been there for me throughout this part of my life's journey. If I do not mention your name, charge it to my mind and not my heart. I thank my parents, Lillian W. Culpepper and Willie L. Battle. I thank my siblings, Donald Ray Harvey, Melvin Harvey, and Telesha Renee Battle. In no particular order, Tracy Pittman, Reshelle Petty, Zobie Davis, Janice Boglin, Margette Wardlaw, Artenze Hall, Shunta Solomon, and Robin Long; I want to thank you for your prayers, listening to me cry, crying with me and for me, bringing over home cooked meals, calling me, texting me, and just being you. Thank you to Tina Greer for mentoring us through this project. Thank you to my partner in this life, Octavian, who is here through thick and thin still loving me; let's continue this ride Boo. Some of you know parts of this story but only ONE being knows it all and he is my Father God. I am so grateful for his continued grace and mercy over my life. I thank him for loving me when I didn't even love myself. This one thing I know for sure...without HIM, I am nothing but with HIM I can do ALL things. - Sandra

Thank you Mom and Dad for the blueprint on how marriage and family is done; it is never written but felt around the dark using faith, love, laughter, and funk music as your guide. For my brothers, who live everyday better than most people I've seen on television; inspire your kids to do as much. My late grandparents, both from the Braxton side and Wood; you are a vast reservoir of strength and possibility that I have yet to emulate. And lastly, to my wife for whom my life I share my heart to under God's blessings; I am in awe of your courage to write this, and share the pain lived, to families everywhere with an empty crib. - Octavian

Introduction

Why is getting pregnant such HARD WORK for me and Suzie Q can get pregnant just like that (snaps finger)? I can't tell you how many times I asked that question. How many times I asked the Lord that question. How many times I cried. How many times I cried out. How many times I blamed myself. How many times I blamed the Lord. How many times I wanted to DIE. YES...I said it. I felt that if I couldn't give birth to a child that I wasn't worthy of life.

A story of infertility, pain, frustration, and loss.   How did we start this journey? Octavian and I were married in 1998. In 2001, we purchased a bigger home and our family and friends were asking when we would be having a baby. We found out that we were pregnant and we were thrilled. I wanted to pour into a baby the love that I never could seem to find for myself; that unconditional, everlasting, overflowing love. I willingly had it to give but needed a baby to give it to, or so I thought.

I told Octavian multiple times that I would give him a divorce. That he deserves a wife that could give him a child. He deserves a family. He is a good man and would make a great father. I didn't want him to feel trapped here with me. YES...I felt that life with me was a trap. Now what does that say? I felt really low. Who out there understands me? But like me, I hope you now understand that your life is ALWAYS worth living. You always have something to give. This test is now my testimony. I pray that it helps someone else along the way.

We pray that this book will open up dialogue and discussion in book clubs, in your homes, in counseling sessions, in churches, in networking groups, on social media, and in all media worldwide.

We have placed discussion breaks throughout the book to encourage that dialogue. Let's start talking.

Sandra's Background:

I am the third child of Lillian Battle and the first child of Willie Battle. I have two older brothers that were bore from my Mom's first marriage. I have a younger sister. We lived most of our life in Battleboro NC, a town with one stop light, no major shopping center and had a railroad running through the middle of it. Our fun days were filled with playing hop scotch, double dutch and kick ball in the middle of the street. My Parents were taught and believed that the only way you would make it in this world was by hard work. Neither of which were afforded the opportunity to complete High School. Dad was raised on a farm and Mom on the brickyard. Back in their younger days, children were your work hands and everyone chipped in to harvest the crops and do the work. School wasn't as important as eating so there were many times that they missed school to stay home to help out. Making enough to pay bills and put food on the table was difficult and it took everything for their families just to make ends meet. Lillian is the bible toting disciplinarian daughter of a Preacher and she always drilled the importance of education. Willie is the hard working, old-fashioned son of a spit fire Father and mild mannered Mother. He worked the same job until he retired. I never went without food, shelter or any of the basic necessities of life. I also never remember them saying the words "I love you" as a kid. They probably never heard it said in their households either. You learn from your parents, whether intentional or not. I believe that they did what they could with what they had. Although it was unspoken, we all loved each other. It was always my intention to be the one to break some of the generational chains in my family...and in my adulthood I am proud to have achieved just that.

My Sister Renee and I were just 10 months apart in age. So many people assumed that we were twins as Momma dressed us alike and we were similar in size. At one time, Renee and I had what I would classify as a normal Sisterly relationship. It became strained approximately nine (9) months after she had her first child at 17 and moved out of our parents' home. I wish it wasn't so because I love my Sister even though we look at life differently. I have reached out in the way that I knew how in attempts to repair our relationship. Sometimes it would seem that we were back on track and then not.

As the dark-skinned one, I never felt pretty enough. I was always compared to my lighter-skinned sister. I would hear people say "Nay is so pretty and Sandy is so smart". I was known as the smart one. I had low self-esteem which led me down the road to poor choices in males. I spent money on men thinking it would make them love me. I would change my hair style, lose weight, and allow them to disrespect me...all in the search for love. I was searching for it but I never knew how it was supposed to feel and because of that I couldn't distinguish between healthy and unhealthy love.

My brothers Donald and Melvin were much older than I was. I remember Donald not being around much and going off to the military at a very young age. Melvin was a Lady's man in High School and a lot of girls would befriend me to ask about him. He has a great personality and was always a sharp dresser. From the beginning I saw that boys were treated differently than girls in our family. I remember my brother having girls over and bringing them into his bedroom. There is no way that would occur with me or my Sister. And my uncertainty of genuine friendships derived from girls befriending me to get to my brother.

Our family enjoyed a modest life. We lived in a house in a neighborhood surrounded by other black families trying to make a better life for themselves. Some of our most memorable times occurred on Christmas morning. The tree was always packed with gifts and we would tear them open with excitement. Getting good grades was a MUST in our house and we all did that. Each of us spent time on the Honor Roll. I graduated third in my class of a group of approximately Ninety Seven (97). I earned a scholarship to NC A&T and it was assumed that I would attend there. As you will read further in this book, I have made many missteps in my life. One of which was not utilizing that scholarship and going to NC A&T in Greensboro NC. I stayed home because I didn't want to leave a boyfriend, so many bad decisions made due to chasing love in all the wrong places. After a failed semester in the local college, I enlisted in the Air Force.

Running won't solve your issues, you just pack them up and take them with you until you fix them. I continued my cycle of bad relationships. My first marriage was to Reggie. We met at the Army Base at the Club where he followed me around like a puppy all night long. He didn't approach me until the end of the night and asked my name. I wasn't attracted to him initially but he seemed nice and drove a nice car. We exchanged information and began dating. After a short courtship, we married on Valentine's Day. Neither of us really knew the other. This was a marriage doomed to fail. And it did...fail I mean. We both were abusive to the other. There was name calling, arguing constantly and then infidelity on his part. I attempted to have a baby thinking this would fix our marriage. It ended in an ectopic pregnancy and I found myself alone in the Hospital. I was devastated but had no clue what a bullet I had dodged. I didn't have the chance to fully grieve the loss of this baby as our marriage was crumbling all around me. Once our marriage became physically violent, I knew I had to escape. I filed for divorce and was relieved once I received the Divorce Decree in my hand.

I was introduced to Octavian by my girl Reshelle AKA Re. She had mentioned this guy to me a couple of times talking about him being "fine." I was intrigued to see who this person was because Re didn't call many guys "fine." One day, we were at the base gym to watch the guys play basketball. On the military base, this was one of our past-times. I had joined the Air Force six years earlier at 19 and was hanging out watching the guys before beginning my work out routine. So while watching the guys play Re said, "There. There he is." I was thinking...HIM? Not saying that he was bad looking but the way all the girls talked about him I was expecting a Morris Chestnut look-alike. I wasn't initially impressed. So we finished watching the game and I went into the cardio room to get on the treadmill. I hated to exercise but in the military you had to maintain a certain weight so I had no choice. I used to be skinny in high school but those days were long gone. After working out, I ran into Octavian again and we caught each other's eye. Now, I have never been known for being shy around a guy. I smiled and he smiled back. After chatting for a quick minute, I asked him if he would be at the NCO Club on Friday night. That's the military base hang out spot. He said that he would and he would see me there. I was celebrating my divorce from Reggie. I just received my signed divorce decree and was going to party hard. Octavian and I were on the dance floor that Friday night dancing to "This is How We Do It" by Montel Jordan and we have been together ever since.

Man's Stigma

The stigma of "What is wrong with her" is always there. You feel the whispers, even if no one is whispering. There is constant pressure. And why is the pressure always on the female? There is this blame game that occurs. It's got to be you. It can't be me. There's no one in my family with infertility issues. So before Octavian agreed to go see the Infertility Specialist, I had to deal with him thinking that this was MY issue and I needed to go to the doctor, NOT him. He shouldn't be taking tests. What for? Even though the doctor said that he needed **both** of us to take tests just to rule out the other, Octavian didn't feel it necessary. We went through this discussion for a year to be exact. This took away precious time that could have been used for resolving our infertility issues. Why do men in general feel this way? Why does society put so much pressure on women when fertility is actually a couple's issue? It is a scientific fact that it takes <u>two</u> beings to produce one. – ***Discussion Break***

Have you experienced this in your journey? _____

How did you deal with it?

_____

_____

Do you agree with my assessment? Why or Why Not?

_____

_____

_____

Chapter 1: Practice Makes Perfect

When you are trying to get pregnant, you are given all kinds of advice. Have sex on your head. Lay in the bed with your legs closed tight all night after he ejaculates in you. Hold your butt up in the air after sex to help the sperm get to your eggs. Do it doggy style. Eat right and take your vitamins. Count your days so you will know when you are ovulating....UGH!!! There is no shortage of people willing to give you their "sure fire" way to get pregnant.

I was 31 and already had experienced an ectopic pregnancy in my first marriage. That means I only had 1 fallopian tube left. I was seeing the infertility specialist for one year before Octavian scheduled his first appointment. The doctor recommended that I have the HSG (Hysterosalpingogram) test. If you've had that done, you know that it is very uncomfortable. A radiographic contrast (dye) is injected into the uterine cavity through the vagina and cervix. The uterine cavity fills with dye and if the fallopian tubes are open, dye fills the tubes and spills into the abdominal cavity. This shows whether the fallopian tubes are open or blocked and whether a blockage is at the junction of the tube and uterus (proximal) or at the other end of the tube (distal). My results came back positive which meant that my remaining tube was unblocked. Awesome news!!!

Octavian went and had a sperm count done. It was determined that his count was low and he required varicocele repair. The doctor recommended surgery, so it was scheduled. This was an outpatient surgery and my Octavian is a very muscular man. After surgery he was still out of it because of the anesthesia, and our house has stairs. I had to get this man up the staircase to the bedroom. Help me Jesus. I used some muscles that I didn't know I had that day. You do what you have to do, don't you? He was out of work for the next three days recovering. His follow up appointment brought great news; his sperm count was now normal. YES!!! We can resume activity.

We had the all clear from our doctors. So it was ON!!! PRACTICE, PRACTICE, PRACTICE!!! And that is what we did too. All the time. We had a four bedroom house and we made sure to christen every room. Oops, did you come visit? Well, we made sure to wash all the sheets before you came over Boo...haha. We did it on the staircase. Ouch, that one hurt my back. We were cooking in the kitchen but no food was being served. We even worked the spin cycle on the washing machine. Oh, the fun we had. We were young and in love. So getting this part done wasn't a problem. That's what the doctor told us to do. Don't stress he said. Don't worry and let it happen is what everyone told us.

A couple of months later...One thing I can count on, besides the tax man, was my period. But this month, I was late. I was cautiously optimistic. I stopped by the pharmacy and picked up a pregnancy test. I was driving fast all the way home. My mind was racing the entire time. I tried not to get my hopes up too high but all the while I was praying that it would be positive. I peed on the stick and vacuumed the carpet to keep me busy for five minutes while the stick would turn pink or blue. I couldn't contain myself as I came back into the bathroom and the stick revealed that I was pregnant.

I was overjoyed. This was truly one of the happiest days of my life. I want the baby to look like me and act like him. I don't want a girl because I did some bad things when I was young and I heard that you get all that back when you have children. Oh Lord, please forgive me for all the wrong that I have done.

I picked up the phone and called Octavian at work. I couldn't wait until he got home to show him the stick. He was just as excited as I was. It was, "Baby how you feel?" "Baby you need something?" "Baby you hungry?" I loved every minute of it...

UNTIL...there was blood, then there was excruciating pain. I was rushed to the hospital where I was informed that I had an ectopic pregnancy. NOT AGAIN!!! REALLY? So what does this mean? I knew what it meant but I was in extreme denial. As the doctor came into my ER room and asked me to sign the document for surgery, I broke down. I almost took the paperwork out of his hand to throw it across the room. That's how mad I was. It wasn't that doctor's fault but I needed someone to blame. The surgery would remove my last remaining fallopian tube. It was the last remaining chance for me to conceive my own baby naturally. I was devastated. I was beyond devastated. NO...WHY...THIS CAN'T BE...WHY US...WHY ME???

I remember Octavian calling my Mom. I really don't remember what happened next. I believe that I block some of the memories that are so painful out of my head. I do remember coming home and no longer being pregnant. I felt empty inside. I remember being numb. I didn't know what was next and if I was willing to stay around to see the end. – *Discussion Break*

Who do you know that has experienced infertility?
_____
_____
_____

Chapter 2: The Best Auntie Ever

I've always showered love on other people's children. I started to do it more after the second ectopic pregnancy happened. I figured if I wasn't going to experience motherhood then I would be the best darn Auntie ever. As a child, I don't recall having any significant relationship with my extended relatives. I wanted to make sure that my nieces and nephews didn't have that same memory of me (breaking that generational chain).

My family rarely have family reunions. To be honest, I don't know a lot about many of my family members. We would only get together during funerals. I haven't been to a funeral in quite a few years now. Not because people haven't died, but because I'd rather remember them as they were the last time I saw them alive. My thinking is to give people their flowers while they are alive because they can't smell them once they are dead. Those Publix Grocery Store commercials where you see the table crowded with family members during the Holidays, that wasn't my reality.

Almost every year Octavian and I would get the kids during Spring Break. Most times it would be Jessica, Ashley, Nisha, Jarvis, Wil, and Rob. Jessica, Ashley, and Nisha are my nieces. Jarvis is Octavian's youngest brother. Wil and Rob are brothers as well as Jarvis' best friends. We had so much fun with them. If we were staying in town we would go to Six Flags, the local amusement park and White Water, the local water park. We frequented Dave & Buster's and watched all the latest movies. There were late nights, early mornings, clothes everywhere, and food all over the place but we looked forward to each visit.

I was so excited as I thought about taking them to the most magical place on earth. Octavian and I discussed it and called to ask permission from all the parents. It was a GO! It was 2000 and we were taking them to Disney World and Universal Studios in Orlando, Florida.

A month before that trip was scheduled to occur, my nephew K.K. who was only 10, was hit by a truck and killed at his school bus stop. He was so excited about this trip and I really wanted to see his little face light up at Disney World. Our family was devastated about losing him. This was a very dark time for each of us. He was a bright ray of light; such an innocent and sweet boy. I remember that he gave the best hugs. I loved his little life. Auntie will always love you Babyboy. RIP.

We contemplated cancelling the trip but didn't want to ruin it for the remaining kids. With so much pain and sorrow, we also wanted to lift the spirits of the other kids. So we went in honor of K.K.

Five days in Orlando with six kids. What were we thinking? We packed up Lewis's van and hit the road. It was a great time, an emotional time, a fun-filled time, and a learning time. The kids played in the pool, they rode on the rides all day long, they ate what they wanted, and everyone enjoyed the trip. Octavian and I needed a vacation after that vacation. We were exhausted AND broke. We really were in over our heads but we would do the same thing again if given the chance.

About five years later, we were blessed enough to take a few of them on their first cruise. They helped to fill our house with love and laughter and we truly enjoyed every experience with them.

They are all adults now but it is so rewarding to hear them speak of what we did with them when they were younger. It warms my heart. I definitely did what I set out to do which was to make sure they knew that Auntie loved them. We pray that our contribution to their childhood will be instrumental in making them better human beings.

We didn't just take in children that were related to us by blood. There were neighborhood kids and friends of relatives. It is funny but to not have children, our house seemed to be the hang out spot for kids. They felt comfortable with us. They felt love in our midst. Octavian is a natural mentor. He is really good at it, sharing his knowledge without being preachy. I am a caregiver and a planner. We make an awesome pair. — *Discussion Break*

Who in your childhood left a grand impression on your life?
_____
_____

What did they do?
_____
_____
_____

Do you try to pay it forward? If so, how?
_____
_____
_____

Chapter 3: In vitro – That Option

So as much as I tried to fight it, those thoughts kept creeping back into my mind. I want a baby. Our baby. A little Sandra and Octavian running around the house. Can we have this dream? Is it truly possible? What are our options?

I started researching and found out about in vitro fertilization. O.M.G. It is soooo expensive. Not only is it expensive - $30,000 per cycle ($20,000 for the procedure/clinic visits and $10,000 for the medication), but there is so much involved. We would have to go to the clinic for multiple visits, use the medication at specific times of the day and night, and both of us would be required to be active participants in this journey. But Lord, we REALLY want this baby. So I checked both of our insurance coverages and would you believe it. In vitro is covered by Octavian's health insurance. SERIOUSLY? Whoop, let's get this party started!!!

I was 33 and scared but here was my chance. I called and scheduled the consultation. We went to the initial appointment and they explained the costs, the procedures, and what we would be in store for during the next couple of weeks. We had to decide if we wanted to commit to this and all that it entailed. We followed our hearts and decided to move forward to schedule our first session with the doctor.

Before we arrived for the first session with the doctor, we received a call from the doctor's office saying that the insurance won't pay upfront but will reimburse. Dang! We had to purchase the medication upfront, that's $10,000. They wanted to know if we wanted to keep our appointment or reschedule. What you need to keep in mind is that these appointments are scheduled by the woman's menstrual cycle. So if we didn't keep this appointment, we would have to wait at least another month to start.

So what do we do? We didn't have $10,000 handy. We are proud and hate to ask for help but this time we couldn't do it on our own. We went to family and no one could help. Thank God for friends that love us like family. We borrowed the money from Dre and Robin with the promise to pay them back once the insurance reimbursed on the claims. They came through without hesitation and for that they will always have a special place in our hearts.

So we started the process. Oh boy. Who knew you could be stuck with a needle so many times? I swear my fingers hurt so bad from them taking my blood almost daily. My ass hurt so badly from those progesterone shots. My thighs hurt so bad from the other hormone shots. My arms hurt so bad because we would switch between my arm and thigh. Octavian would give me a shot twice daily. I hate the site of needles so he gave them to me. If I never saw another needle again, it would be too soon. This was not a pleasant experience. In the beginning Octavian enjoyed inflicting pain on me with those needles but after a while even Octavian started to feel bad for me. This went on for three weeks. But the day that they harvested the eggs was a good day. We got good news that they harvested quite a few and the ones that were harvested were of good quality. Because Octavian had previously had surgery for low sperm count, the doctor suggested that we also have the ICSI procedure done. That's where they manually inject the egg with the sperm for a better success rate. We followed the doctor's orders to a T. A few days later, they called with the good news that we had 3 fertilized eggs. YIPPY! SUCCESS!

When we went in for the procedure to get the eggs inseminated, it was suggested that we place all three eggs back into my uterus as there was a chance that only one would take. I was happy and a little nervous at the same time. We were sent home with the instructions to rest which is exactly what we did. Our next appointment would be to find out if the pregnancy is a viable one. I came into the doctor's office alone and took the pregnancy test. They would call me later with the results. That was the longest day EVER!!! The phone rang at work around 4:30 p.m. and a voice on the other end said, "You're pregnant."

It seems that as soon as I hung up the phone I started feeling sick. I'm not sure if that was in my mind or not. Soon after, it definitely wasn't in my mind. I had THE WORST case of morning sickness. If only I knew then what I know now. If you are experiencing terrible morning sickness, try peppermint oil. Put a dab of it in your palm and sniff.

When we were finally able to see the ultrasound, they realized why. All three eggs took...OH MY! We are going to be parents to triplets. Help us somebody.

We picked up the phone and called the world. And I mean the ENTIRE world. Everybody knew that we were pregnant. We were happy and this is what we prayed for. Be careful what you pray for and be ready for it when it comes. This pregnancy wasn't what it was cracked up to be for me though. I was sick as a dog. I couldn't keep anything down. I mean nothing. Water came back up. Crackers came back up. Air came back up. I was miserable. I smelled everything. My senses were so hyper. I couldn't sleep because I was uncomfortable lying down. I was uncomfortable sitting up. I don't know what these kids were in there doing but they were wreaking havoc on me. I lost so much weight. Even though I was pregnant, my clothes were hanging off of me. I remember scaring Octavian to death when I got up in the middle of the night to go to the refrigerator and fainted. All he heard was me hitting the floor. When I came to, I didn't know what had happened.

We went to the doctor and asked if there was something, anything that they could do. Nothing that they suggested helped. I worked in a Call Center and couldn't be at the desk throwing up. So I called in sick. I was missing work. I thought that short-term disability would cover me as a high-risk pregnancy but unfortunately it was denied by the insurance company. Even with signed documentation from my physician they denied the claim. I felt like, why do I even have insurance if it doesn't help when I need help? This experience changed my feeling about insurance and the fact that they are in business to make money, not to make sure you are okay. I was a union employee but hadn't been on my job long enough to receive full sick pay. I had been out for a couple of weeks and was receiving half pay and received notice that either I come back to work or risk losing my job. As if this news wasn't bad enough, Octavian came home and told me that he had been terminated from his job. We are pregnant with triplets, borrowed money from friends to get pregnant, about to be behind on our bills because I've only been getting half pay, Octavian lost his job, and I'm being told to come back or lose mine. Marinate on that for a second.

How quickly can the brightest time of your life turn into the darkest time in your life? I'm used to having control or at least thinking that I have control. I have absolutely no control right now and I feel like there is no one that can help us. I miscarried that night. A very dark time followed this. I still blame myself. I am disappointed that I didn't have enough faith to carry me through. There was a period of time that I strayed away from the church after this occurred. I placed blame on a lot of things; on not having the proper support system, on myself, on God. It was a very difficult time for me.

We would attempt two additional cycles in the next two years. During which I also tried acupuncture as I was told that it would "open up" my uterus. If you are keeping count, that's approximately $90,000 that we spent on this option. The money for the last two cycles came from withdrawals from my 401K. Neither of the last two cycles produced a pregnancy. Each IVF cycle would leave me feeling defeated, drained, emotional, and hormonal. I was being pumped with hormones during each of these cycles and any woman will tell you we are already hormonal enough without being pumped with additional amounts of it. I know during this time I was moody, bitchy, mad, and depressed. I'm sure there were many times that I lashed out at the people that cared most about me and that I cared about. **Hurt people, hurt people. I was hurt.** Keep in mind that during all of this I'm still being asked "When are you guys going to have a baby?" "Have you talked to your doctor?" "What did the doctor say?" "Why haven't you had a baby yet?" Looking back I know it was God that kept me sane. – ***Discussion Break***

Have you ever dealt with insurance issues that were detrimental to your finances?

_____

_____

How important is your faith to you?

_____

_____

Chapter 4: I Couldn't Do Baby Showers

Oh my! Just like a single woman and weddings...I felt that everywhere I looked I saw a pregnant belly. Everyone I knew was pregnant. Their friend was pregnant. A co-worker was pregnant. A neighbor was pregnant. So here comes the baby shower invitations. What am I supposed to do? It is rude not to go, right?

Ya'll, during this time I couldn't look at baby clothes without crying. I couldn't walk down an aisle in the store with baby food without getting emotional. Hey, I'm only human. Yes, I was happy for her when she got pregnant but I just couldn't muster up the might to go to the baby shower. So I would make up an excuse not to go. I always had something else to do. I would always send a gift though. I love those gift registries. I didn't have to go to the store, just shop online. Pick it out, pay for it, they ship it, DONE.

It had nothing to do with her. It was me. I was dealing with my own stuff. But guess what? It's okay that I chose not to participate in the event. Always remember to choose you. Choose what's best for you where you are in your life. We always get so caught up in making sure everyone else is happy, making sure everyone else is okay but are we okay?

During this time, it was not okay for me to show up at another person's shower and possibly not show them the kind of happiness that I did feel for them hidden in the sorrow that I felt for myself. I wasn't sure which they would see and if it would be misunderstood. To avoid any miscommunication, I skipped it.

Chapter 5: Adoption – Final Option

A couple of years before we had attended an introduction meeting at Bethany Christian Services Adoption Agency to listen to the adoption services that they offer. We met many other couples going through similar situations that we were going through. We took the package home and sat it on the coffee table. I don't believe we were ready to move forward with that choice just yet because the paperwork never got filled out and we never followed through.

Although the cost for the open adoption of an African American baby is cheaper than the average cost of adopting a Caucasian baby, it still cost between $12,000 and $15,000. I tell you what, we are going bankrupt in the attempts to be parents. Something that most people take purely for granted. Not only would an open adoption be taxing on our wallet, it also allows for the birth mother to remain in contact with the family. You get to choose how the communication is done but you do agree to remain in contact with this birth mother. You are also picked by the birth mother. For that to happen, you have to put together a package of pictures, letters, and information about yourself for the birth mother to look at in hopes that you would be chosen. Now think about this for a minute. Not only are you agreeing to allow the birth mother to remain in your life via letters, pictures, or other forms of communication, you are at the mercy of being chosen by your pictures, letters, etc. AND you have to pay thousands of dollars for this privilege. Process that.

I wasn't sure if I was okay with the birth mother remaining a part of our lives. You hear stories all the time of the birth family showing up on the adoptive parents' doorstep asking for their baby back and confusing the heck out of the child. My God. Who wants that?

We did receive emails from some of the other couples that attended the same meeting with updates on their adoptions. Each time I saw an email, I would think that we needed to DO SOMETHING. I was happy for them but sad for us. Time waits for no one and we aren't getting any younger. For me, age was a huge factor because I made it one. I put a limit on it. I told Octavian that if we didn't get pregnant or adopt before I turned 40 that it was going to be taken off the table. In my mind, I didn't want to be the woman going to the daycare being asked if that was my grandchild instead of my child. I didn't want to be 50 years old with an infant child. I didn't want to die while my child was still in high school. All of those were thoughts of mine. I didn't want to do that to the child or myself.

We heard from Aunt Maida, who is a high school teacher that one of her students is pregnant with her second child and not financially able to take care of either child. She wanted to know if we were interested in meeting this girl to discuss adoption. We said OF COURSE. So we scheduled a weekend to drive to Virginia where they were located to meet this young lady having no idea what we would encounter.

Upon meeting her and her son (he wasn't even 2 yet), we immediately fell in love with the boy. He was adorable. She was what you would expect, young and ignorant to life. We ended up spending most of the day with her. We ate at Golden Coral and talked to her while trying to figure out what she wanted out of life. What we didn't realize is that she was enamored with the Mercedes Benz that we were driving. She had already assumed that she could "get something" out of this deal. While we were thinking of helping her, she was thinking of getting one over on us. Sad, but true.

On the way to take her home, we stopped by the grocery store to pick up a couple of healthy food items to make sure she was eating right for the baby and stopped by the post office to purchase stamps as she had promised to write to keep us updated on the health of the baby. We left her thinking we may possibly adopt her son and the new baby (a daughter). That would make our family complete while allowing her to follow her dreams in life knowing that her children were being cared for by a loving family. What a great feeling we had.

Well, those thoughts changed as soon as we received her first letter after our visit. The letter was supposed to update us on the status of her doctor visits but instead the letter was a "request" for rent money. In the letter, she went on to say that if she didn't get the money, her and her son would be out on the street with nowhere to go. I wrote her back asking what did she mean by her letter and reminding her that we had an agreement to adopt her baby not to pay her bills. We refused to buy a baby. No matter how cute it was. This was heartbreaking for us. Not just because of the baby she was carrying but because we were extremely fond of the son that she already had and really couldn't care for. What would become of these children? My God. That was our last communication. We never heard back from her. We were told by Aunt Maida that she had delivered the baby girl and dropped out of high school. As we feared, both children ended up in the system. No family members stepped up to the plate to take them and she was too busy running after the baby's father which we understand to be a narcotics dealer.   I still wonder about those beautiful kids and the life they could have had with us. What a shame.

Fast forward two years after that happened. Mary Nell called saying that she heard about this young lady that is pregnant, in college, and looking to give the baby up for adoption. Knowing that we have already been down this road, I was hesitant. Mary Nell is a dear military friend and I trust her implicitly. She knows of this girl by way of her adopted daughter's father who is a counselor of young people at his church. I got him on the phone and talked to him extensively as well. The Birth Mom is a church going girl that is now pregnant and unmarried. We all have sinned and come short of God's glory.

When I finally get the chance to talk to this young lady on the phone, she and I hit it off immediately. It had gotten to where we were talking on the phone daily. Most times not even about the pregnancy. She needed guidance in her life and I took it as a chance to impart my knowledge onto her. She was 21 and wanted a lot out of life but had no clue how to go about getting it. I shared my experiences with her. I did this from a genuine heart because if I was in her situation I would want someone to do that for me. I told her many times to think it over and make sure that the adoption is what she wanted to do because she would have to live with this decision for the rest of her life. She told me that she knew she wanted her son to have a better life than she could provide and she could tell that I would be an awesome mom.

After weeks of talking on the phone to this young lady every day and believing that she was sincere we hired a lawyer to handle the adoption and advise on the legal process. The lawyer informed us of the three day waiting period in the state of North Carolina, where the young lady resided. Every state has different laws so be sure you know the laws of the state in which you plan to adopt. This means that she has three days to change her mind after the baby is born. Are you kidding me? **It's the law.** What many people don't realize is that the laws DO NOT protect the adoptive parents. We have NO rights. We are at the mercy of the birth mother. It doesn't matter how invested we are in the process or the baby, more times than not we end up on the losing end.

The lawyer gave us some paperwork to take with us when we visited her to get her and her boyfriend to sign to give their consent and specify their desire to give the baby up for adoption. In my mind I'm thinking...Here we go again. We arrange a visit. On the phone with her, I requested that we meet ALL parties involved to make sure that we were all on the same page. I asked that their parents join us in this meeting as well. Especially because this relationship was not condoned by the parents, although they were still seeing each other. See, she was white and he was black. He was also in college and only 20 years old.

So Octavian and I drive to Fayetteville. We met the girl and boyfriend at the doctor's office. She wanted us to come to her appointment in hopes that we could see the ultrasound. The doctor allowed me to go with her back in the room and listen to the heartbeat which was very strong. The baby is healthy, the doctor proclaims. This girl and her boyfriend were very nice and respectful. They were clean cut and you could tell that they both came from decent families. They were both in college and working part-time jobs. After the doctor's appointment, we went out to lunch at Olive Garden. We enjoyed their company but I inquired about the whereabouts of their parents. The young man stated that his parents were too busy and couldn't join us. The young lady stated that we would get to meet her parents later.

This gave us pause but they both signed the paperwork from the lawyer's office willingly and in front of a notary. We took this action as a show of faith. We had to keep moving forward. Before we left to come back home, the young lady's parents invited us over to their home. How gracious I thought. They didn't mind that we know where they live? They had a modest home as a military family with a working background. I related to them especially being from the military. They treated us like old friends. The young lady's mother and I began communicating as we exchanged numbers as well. She said she would be sure to call us first when her daughter went into labor. The ride home was a good one. We were both upbeat and happy about the situation. We believed this was our baby.

Now, we would tell everyone. We decided to name our son Andrew. We decorated the nursery. I had been looking at this nursery set in JC Penney's for months now. I can finally buy it and put it in the empty room upstairs. And that I did. It had a safari theme with beautiful earth tones. I went to Hobby Lobby and bought the cutest wooden animal cut-outs and meticulously placed them on the wall. We registered just like all parents do and had a baby shower. Margette threw it at our house and so many of our friends showed up with beautiful gifts for Andrew. We were overwhelmed with the response. Our family and friends that couldn't make the shower were sending gifts in the mail especially my Cousin Robin. She really was blessing Andrew. Our military friends J.T. and Renee shipped us a beautiful rocker. This baby had EVERYTHING!!! We had diapers for newborn up to size two (2). I think we covered all the bases. My Mother-in-law Lucia gave me this Nursery Rhyme book that I couldn't wait to read from every night before putting Andrew to bed. The nursery was absolutely beautiful. I would go in there some days and just be, just stare, just pick up something and sniff around. I was so happy. I was ready to receive this blessing.

And so the phone rang in the middle of night. "She's in labor," is what her Mom told me. I already had the diaper bag packed and ready for this call. Octavian and I jumped out of bed, took our showers and got in the car. The car seat was already in the car too. We drove to Fayetteville and checked into the Hotel. We figured we would be here for three days as the final paperwork couldn't be signed until after the 3-day waiting period. I called my job to notify them that my leave would begin today. I had applied for a 6-week leave of absence and been approved. They all knew the situation and were overjoyed for us. My heart was beating so fast. I was nervous, scared, excited all of those at the exact same time. We drove up to the hospital. We went into her hospital room and she was still in labor. Her parents were there and they were glad to see us. That was a relief. I'm still afraid that something will go wrong. They asked the doctor if we could go into the delivery room with her and were told No. The boyfriend goes into the delivery room instead. She delivers a beautiful baby boy. As soon as they are wheeled back into the room, she asks the nurse to let us hold the baby. Octavian and I both hold Andrew. I get a picture of Octavian holding him. He has that proud Dad look on his face.

Then the hospital door swings open and the entire environment changes. The boyfriend's family arrives. They walk in and instead of speaking to everyone in the room, they look around and see me, Octavian, and the young lady's parents and walk right over to the baby who was lying in the bassinet. They proceeded to pick the baby up and say that they are so glad that their baby is here. Jesus, here we go. They put the baby down and then speak in a loud tone "and who are they" while pointing at me and Octavian.

The young lady's parents state that "they are the adoptive parents."

The boyfriend's mother then states that "ain't nobody taking my grandchild nowhere." If I had a thermostat on my forehead it would have popped, that's how hot I was at that moment. Where the heck have they been? I've asked about them for months but never heard back. We drove all the way here to meet you guys and you didn't show up. Well, here they are and it's about to get ugly.

They must have picked up the phone and called the whole dang family because the hospital room door kept opening, each time with more members of his family. Each one coming into the room giving Octavian and I the evil eye and kissing on the baby. What is going on here? We are not the enemy. Where were you guys when these kids were going through this pregnancy? If you were so supportive, they would have never reached out to a couple of strangers to ask us to take care of their baby. So don't look at me like I did something wrong. As a matter of fact, I'm the only one trying to do something right. Right for the future of this child.

As the room continued to fill, Octavian and I walked out to call our lawyer's office. I wanted to get legal counsel. I explained what was going on at the Hospital. Our Lawyer's assistant said unfortunately, if she doesn't sign the paperwork in three days we would be leaving that Hospital empty handed. Are you serious? After all we have been through. Where is the justice in this situation? Does anyone care about the rights of the adoptive parents? We have feelings too. We've spent all of this money. Our families are sitting by the phone waiting to hear the good news. All of our friends are waiting for us to come home with Andrew. Who the hell cares about us???

After stepping away to call the lawyer and getting a bite to eat, we returned to the hospital room. Immediately we knew it was a done deal. She had changed her mind. The boyfriend's Mom was sitting on the edge of her bed while she was holding the baby. They were both smiling and looking at the baby. She is not going to sign the papers. We hugged her parents and told them goodbye. They begged us to stay but we've been through this before. When you see the writing on the wall, you don't deny it. As painful as it was, we had to accept it and leave. I truly don't recall the drive back to Atlanta. I called our parents and a couple of close friends to tell them what had happened and then I shutdown. My heart was aching. I didn't know if I was coming or going. I'm glad Octavian was driving because I'm not sure if I would have known which way to drive. I was distraught. The backseat held an empty car seat. The house had a fully decorated nursery that would not have an occupant. In my mind I'm screaming, "What in the world? What are we doing wrong? Are we bad people? Why does this keep happening to us?"

The room that I would just go and spend hours being in became the room that I avoided like the plague. It was difficult for me to walk past the room. I shut the door so I wouldn't see a glimpse of anything inside. I had signed up for a couple of baby sites and booklets and offers started coming in the mail. Frequent reminders of what we failed to bring home. Although it wasn't my fault, I thought back over all of my conversations with her to see if I said something wrong or if I missed a sign that she gave early on that she would do this to us. I racked my brain and couldn't figure it out. There is no way of knowing. And you wonder why more people don't adopt or why they fly over to China/Africa/Russia and bring babies back when there are so many children here in need of a loving home. Adoptive parents take all of the risk in this country. The laws suck for us.

The nursery door remained closed for years. I would go in there every now and then and have a good cry. We would get phone calls about others who were interested in giving their child up for adoption but we were no longer interested in going through the process. Yes, we still had the desire of being parents but not the desire of experiencing any more pain. For me, the fear of more pain became larger than the desire to parent. – *Discussion Break*

Have you attempted adoption before? If so, how was your experience?

_____

_____

Do you understand the adoption laws in your state?

_____

_____

Did you realize how difficult adoption is?

_____

_____

Would you have continued attempting to adopt given what we went through?

_____

_____

Chapter 6: Cookie Braxton, Unconditional Love Found

Cookie, my Pekinese Poodle (Peekapoo) mix dog believed that I birthed her. She would bite you if you told her otherwise...LOL. I wasn't raised with pets so the fact that I have a dog is funny to the rest of my family, especially because I was always afraid of them. This fear came from ignorance. We have a family portrait of my Mom, Dad, sister, myself, and two brothers. In the portrait, I am crying. I asked my Mom why I was crying in that family portrait and she said because there was a dog in the studio when we took the picture. I had never been around dogs and therefore had no knowledge of them. Octavian told me that I needed to spend time around dogs to get over my fear. In 2001 our neighbor across the street named Lynn had the cutest dog named Coco (a chocolate Peekapoo). She was a small thing and I figured she couldn't hurt me. I would go to their house and play with her in the yard every day after work. Lynn told me that the breeder that she got Coco from had one doggie left and would sell her to me if I was interested. This dog was considered the "runt" of the litter so she would sell her for $225. I immediately said yes.

That's how we got Cookie. The love of my life. When we first got her, she could fit in the palm of my hand. She would run away from me though and I didn't understand why. Octavian told me to give her time. It took three days and then she would run to me when I came home from work. It was the best feeling ever. I would scold her and she would cower for a moment, and then she'd be jovial again, running right back into my arms. What is this? I've never experienced it before. It was unconditional love; something I'd been looking for my entire life and I found it in this doggie.

Cookie was my twin, this dog had the same characteristics as me. She was definitely a Diva. She was finicky about her food. She didn't just eat anything. She didn't like a dirty bowl of water; nope, her water must be clean. She was also gas happy. As soon as she heard the keys jingle, she was ready to go for a ride in the car. She enjoyed putting her head out the window and letting the wind blow directly in her face. That's my girl. So she's the closest thing to having a child of my own. She called me Mommy, in her doggie voice. Having her around was a tremendous help during each infertility struggle. It's like she could sense my hurt and pain. She would cuddle up beside me on the bed to remind me that she was here and it was gonna be okay. That's my Cookie. Yep, I have experienced motherhood; albeit to a sweet dog but motherhood just the same.

Known for her beautiful fur, Cookie's fur started thinning and she was no longer able to leap onto the bed in one long bound like she used to. Of course, we knew she was getting older and so we just attributed it to old age. Unfortunately, it was more than just that. After many tests by the Vet it was determined that our beloved Cookie had Cushing's disease at the age of 11. She had lost so much weight, she no longer had any energy and just wasn't the same doggy. We made the decision to put her down at the age of 12 after seeing she was in pain. I held her and felt her last heartbeat. Now THAT was the hardest thing that I've had to do in my entire life which is saying a lot. She passed two weeks after my birthday in October. We went on a cruise for my birthday that year. I started not to go because I felt that she was close to the end. I really regret going and leaving her. That is the only cruise that I have been on that didn't enjoy. I wish I had spent those last days with Cookie because I can never get those days back.

After Cookie passed, I walked around in a daze for weeks. I was just trying to make it from sun up to sun down. I was depressed. I had lost my baby. Once again I felt empty. I was truly uncertain how I would keep going forward. Cookie was my comforter and my confidant. I told her things that I would never say aloud to another person and she would just give me doggie kisses. No judgement, just love.

After declaring that I would never get another dog because I didn't want to go through the pain of losing one again, I find myself looking at puppies. I didn't want to go through life without that unconditional love that I felt from Cookie. We now have Kali, a beautiful brown and white Cocker Spaniel. She has her own personality which is totally opposite of Cookie. It is so funny at times how different that they are. She has brought her own brand of joy back into the house and we welcome that. – **Discussion Break**

Do you have a pet? If so, what do you have and what is its name?

_____

_____

_____

Have you experienced the therapeutic effect of a pet in your life?

_____

_____

_____

Chapter 7: It's All My Fault

Eighteen is considered the legal age of adulthood in this Country. Although I thought I knew everything at that age, I didn't know a damn thing. I was running wild. I had multiple sex partners. I wasn't employed. I didn't have any money and was still living under my parent's roof. I was a confused child thinking that I was grown. I didn't have a clue.

Then, it happens. You play with fire, you are bound to get burned. I'm a dumb teenager with no way of supporting myself...and pregnant. Who's going to inform my parents? Heck, not me, remember they are very strict and the last thing they want is a pregnant daughter under their roof with no job, no husband and a bleak future. Well, it doesn't take long for them to figure it out as I was consistently running to the bathroom throwing up my guts. So now what? I'm a confused child in an adult situation and the worst part is that I'm not sure who the Father is. I cheated on the guy I was dating during NC A&T's Homecoming. We all were up there partying, having a good time and my fast butt was testing new waters. Not only was I sleeping around, I didn't use protection.

I called my boyfriend to tell him the news. The crazy thing is we just had an argument where I revealed that I hadn't been faithful. I did that to get back at him when really all it did was create a bigger mess for me. I did lots of stupid things during this time. Didn't I say that eighteen shouldn't be considered the legal age of adulthood? I thought I knew everything but I didn't know jack. Well my boyfriend said what you would expect him to say "How do I know that it's mine?" That was a legitimate question of which I really didn't have the answer.

So, feeling like I had nowhere to turn, I made a decision that no teenager should be able to make. I had an abortion. I still remember how I felt that day so vividly. It was an empty feeling inside that I had never experienced before in my life but would unfortunately feel again. I wouldn't wish that on my worst enemy. It is the one thing that I regret most in my life.

So this is why I can't conceive. I'm being punished by God for committing the ultimate sin. I don't blame HIM for punishing me. I would too. Why do I deserve this happiness now? This is the conversation that I was having on the inside. But the truth is, God wasn't punishing me. I had asked for forgiveness years before from HIM. What I needed to do now was forgive myself in order to move forward. Not once did Octavian blame me (due to my past) for our inability to conceive. I did enough of that for the both of us. There are so many others that have had this experience and feel unworthy due to what society says. Don't do that to yourself. He without sin, cast the first stone.

Without therapy, counseling sessions and my Faith, I'm certain that I would have lost my mind. I have been to multiple counselors during different times in this journey. I would go until I start to feel as though I have a handle on things. Anytime I start to feel as though I am losing grip, I schedule an appointment. I don't know why but it is so much easier to pour out your heart to a total stranger. Maybe because you don't feel as if they are judging you for the way you feel or for the things you did. They are unbiased participants just giving you some tools to help you maneuver through difficulty. Keeping this kind of grief, pain, and anger in can become consuming and can affect every area of your life. Talking to a counselor helped me deal with my feelings in healthy ways and showed me when I was not dealing with them.

The true sign of a strong person is when they recognize that they need help and ask for it.

What I do not understand is why there is a stigma on seeking professional help/counseling/therapy in the black community? So many of our family members are in need of this. There are generational curses that need to be broken. A first step to this is seeking professional help. - *Discussion Break*

When have you used counseling/therapy to help you through a difficult time?

_____

_____

Do you also feel that there is a stigma on seeking professional help?

_____

_____

Does your family have generational curses that you would like to see destroyed? What are they? A generational curse is something that is done generation after generation that has a detrimental effect on your future in any way.

_____

_____

_____

_____

_____

Chapter 8: Acceptance

None of us know exactly what is in store for us in this life. But whatever we are given, we should cherish. Octavian and I enjoy the blessing of having each other. We have our own little family consisting of two human family members and a doggie. We are each other's best friend and love each other immensely. Either of us could have easily decided to go our separate ways during the difficult times. Instead, we decided to honor our vows. We know that life together is so much better than life apart.

We look on the bright side. We have the freedom to do whatever we want to do. Traveling is one of the things we love to do. We go on a cruise every other year. We've celebrated an anniversary in Hawaii, birthdays in Jamaica, Las Vegas, and New York City. We will get on the road and spend a long weekend on one of the beaches of Florida or South Carolina. We even got Cookie into it. She had her own luggage and would get excited when she saw me packing it. She would come with us to the Blue Ridge Mountains when we rented cabins there. She absolutely loved it. Becoming the owners of The Braxton Agency was a natural progression.

When I found out that one of my nieces was pregnant, we had yet to enter the Nursery to take it down. Of course I'm going to give her whatever she can use. She's having a girl so I gave her all of the non-gender baby items. Then I found out that a co-worker's wife was having a boy so I packed up the rest and took it to work one day. I told him to come with me to the parking deck and unloaded my trunk into his car. He was in tears with gratitude as he didn't know our story (which I shared while unpacking the trunk). I was able to bless two babies with that nursery. Now **THAT** was a good day! (In my Ice Cube voice)

Chapter 9: The NK (No Kids) Couple Label

As we get older, it becomes more difficult to find couples to spend quality time with. We enjoy going out to dinner, to the movies, to a house party. We like to have fun like everyone else, but for whatever reason it seems that we don't get invited over as often as couples with kids. We would hear, after the fact, that so and so had a party. I don't think people realize that they discriminate against couples without kids. We are perfectly good enough to ask to support your Girl Scout Cookies, purchase your Christmas wrapping paper for the school fundraiser, or to donate monies to your child's field trip but we're not the ones you think of when you have a get together at your house. That's not cool.

Octavian and I are both in our forties but usually end up hanging out with people much older. Most of which have grown children that have left the house and who are ready to experience life again, or ones that are more financially stable and enjoy traveling as much as we do. Either way, we are happy to have a few couples that we call friends.

Some people use their children as an excuse to stop living their own lives. A happy parent is a better one. So why aren't you enjoying your life while raising your child? Don't lose your identity in rearing children. It doesn't have to only be about going to the playground. You can have some grown up time too. We know some people that have had children and haven't been out with adults since. Hire a babysitter. Get out of the house sometime. Having a child should add to your life experience, not take away from it.

Chapter 10: Shining Bright

Through all of this, I have found my strength in my Faith. I am not walking on the edge about to fall off. I love seeing pictures of your kids and enjoy hearing about what's going on with them.   Of course, I have days where I still get emotional but I'm good. Being human means that not all days will be good ones. You have the power to make your days good though. Your mindset, your attitude, and your goals are all determining factors. I choose to be positive. I choose to improve myself. I choose to be around those that are doing the same.

I am very pleased with my life right now. I'm sharing my life with my loving husband and my sweet pooch. We are blessed beyond measure. There is no doubt in my mind that both of my parents love me and I love them. I thank God every day that they are both still alive and well and that he is keeping them in their right mind. I talk to them often and we make sure to say "I love you" to each other on the phone and when we see each other. Don't wait for change to occur, be the change that you want. I am the first person in my immediate family to graduate with a Bachelor's degree and I also now have a Master's degree. I am an Entrepreneur with my own Travel Agency and Jewelry boutique, and I am a Certified Project Manager. Since becoming a Business Owner, I have been exposed to a Circle of people that motivate, support and inspire me. I am very thankful for this.

Writing this book is a huge accomplishment. It has been truly a blessing and it almost didn't happen. I was scheduled to attend a Boss Lady Business Women Event (If you are a Business Owner, attending Networking Events is essential). The devil kept trying to keep me from attending. I had every excuse in the book NOT to go. My head started hurting, I had nothing to wear, it was a long drive. One thing that I know for sure is that the Lord speaks to me in a still quiet voice and when He does, I listen. I heard a voice say that you will miss your blessing if you don't get up and go tonight.

The very first person I met at the Event was Donna, another military veteran. She is a ball of energy and a breath of fresh air. She was telling me about this organization of women veterans (Women Veterans Interactive) that do good things in the community as well as help each other with their Business ventures. I was definitely interested in being a part of that organization(now a lifetime member...whoohoo!). She mentioned that she had written a book. Then here comes another ball of energy hugging Donna. Her name is Kim and she went on to say that she was writing her second book(WOW!). These Ladies showed me so much love that night and it was the first time I had set eyes on either of them. Before the night was over, I reconnected with Tina who I found out was teaching a writing seminar. Writing a book had never crossed my mind. After these interactions, it was clear as day to me. I am supposed to write a book. But about what Jesus? Of course...the most profound journey that I have taken in my life, our struggles with infertility.

I pray that this manuscript has touched you in a positive way. It has definitely been a cathartic release for me as I open myself and share a very personal piece of me with you in the hopes of providing a view, some cheer and some light. We (women) may not all have physical babies but we all are still mothers and therefore mothering. This book is one of my babies.

Chapter 11: The Male View

Contribution by Octavian

There was a time that I was excited to have a child; whether it was my own or the opportunity to raise another when their family didn't have the means, or love to do it themselves. I used to envy the loving and powerful influence my father and mother played in me and my two siblings' lives growing up. Hell, I still do I would suppose, and I wanted to instill that nurturing purpose for our family. When I met my Sandra and eventually married; I knew that I found someone who shared the same understanding on what it will take to raise our child.

I look at my parents now as they are in their 60's and see a dynamic duo who super-powered a relationship with us of trust and expectation. More so since we are children of color, in the wake of a burgeoning teenage concept of civil equality amongst Americans. Raising three precocious young black kids in a less than forgiving world during the craziness of the 1980's and 90's must have been terrifying. Being the oldest of the three, I had a panoramic view through the years of how they raised us and gave us a wonderful childhood despite our setbacks. I could honestly say, in my opinion, that my brothers and I were the last decent generation to fail numerously, in almost every conceivable way, and still come out to win in life in our respective lives. Our parents gave us just enough rope so we could learn to pull ourselves up and do the right thing the next time around. Between my brothers and I, as we were growing up (besides the usual teenage hi-jinks of rebellion and misadventure), we had rap sheets that included arson, shoplifting, black marketing, fighting (and a lot of it), and breaking curfew. I know, that last one raises an eyebrow or two compared to the other list of ills we contributed to our parent's worries and society at large. Consider that we grew up on a military base in a small town called Aschaffenburg, Germany, for eight years and that as Americans we were expected to honor our host country with decorum and civility, which breaking curfew would be right up there with burning the basement down with matches and Popsicle sticks. We weren't bad kids we just did supremely stupid things that pointed the question of whether we were going to grow up to be accomplished in any way that did not include stints in the pen. We did well in school and participated in community functions and sports, but that wild streak kept us in trouble at times. I guess it was to be expected, but what I didn't count on, to make my point, was how these experiences shaped our world views later on in life. Like, how our parents raised us. Sure they sometimes grounded us, withheld allowance, or beat the brakes off of us at times, but it was out of love. They wanted more from us than we knew or cared to find in ourselves. They wanted to fulfill an unspoken promise to their parents, grandparents, and everyone in our extended family (it takes a village, right) that we will take their thoughts, fears, triumphs, strengths, love and soul beyond their limits.

That is what good parents want for their children, right? You want to give them structure, and the challenges to prosper, whatever the difficulty. You are to be the extension of their lineage; the Simba to their Mustafa, so to speak (if you haven't seen Disney's Lion King by now, we have nothing to talk about). Why else are you part of a family? Parenting is a horror movie until the child reaches adulthood; you are just hoping that your kid doesn't trip over unseen obstacles as the killer looms over them to deliver the death blow. Once you get older and you realize what your parents were trying to do, it's a comedy full of laughs and hilarious bits of nostalgia that never gets old. My parents got the best of both worlds, and they are proud of every one of those moments, for good or ill, for that is what tests our resolve growing up. We were a family, taking on the world. I wanted that for me and my wife, too. Life denied us that privilege to have what my parents gave me and my brothers; what my grandparents fostered in my parents.

I am a product of the past. A living representation of a long loving history and active ideals that my parents have instilled in me ever since I was born in a little town called Farmville, Virginia. I am the first grandchild of the late Lucille and Walter Wood, and the first born of Lewis Braxton and Lucia Wood, who at a young age (20 years and 15 years, respectively) in 1974, had no idea what their lives counted for back then, but they did know unequivocally that I was the priority.

The game changer as it were, was that my parents needed to re-evaluate their lives. I imagine most parents go through such revelation. When you realize that the stakes just went up, what do you do? Luckily, my parents weren't alone in the love they had to offer me, and allowed my grandparents a solid hand in my foundation. My mother was much too young, unmarried, and unequipped to solely raise me on her own; she was still in High School. My father, a strapping 170 pound lad as he would put it, did not have the means to support me working in the town that time forgot. Seriously, Farmville, Virginia, was one of those towns that was stuck in the late 1960's for the better part of 20 years. If my father and mother decided to stay and raise me there, I don't think the family structure would have stayed intact or grown well. As it were, they all had a plan; I was to stay with my grandparents in Farmville, while my mother finished high school to pursue her degree at Virginia Commonwealth University; my father, however, joined the United States Army. I cannot put into words what

Lucille and Walter Wood has been for my life. They played as surrogates while my parents gathered themselves to task, and raised me as their own until the time was right to be my parent's responsibility. I know regardless, that I was loved and heavily favored by the amount of support my parents received from Lucille and Walter, and by extension, the rest of my family and their friends.

Everyone had a hand in raising me (again, it took a village) but my grandparents laid the groundwork for my domestic education. Maybe it was the excitement of another baby in the house, or the prospect of an empty nest to soon come. My mother was the second youngest of seven children in the small, three bedroom house where discipline, hard work, education, and church was the standard. A big family that extends beyond just the Wood name; we are called Spraggs, Redds, and Hurt just name a few, but all, in one way or another, had their hands on me which played a part in my eventual development.

Lucille was nurturing and kind, whose smile sung me a song whenever she held me...I see her in my mind's eye to this day and I find it hard not to cry since her passing in 2007. Walter, on the other hand was a hard, proud man who taught me hard work and discipline. I marveled at how he got up every morning an hour before the crack of dawn, without an alarm clock, to work various jobs to keep the house afloat, from the dawn's light of the moon to the setting of the evening sun.

Lucille worked various jobs herself, most notably of which, that stuck out in my mind, was the little hairdresser shop that she owned. I tell you, it was no bigger than a walk-in closet but everyone near and far came to get their hair done under that little roof, and I was her little helper.

With Walter, I learned to shoot a gun, fish, can foods, dumpster dive, pull crops, you name it. That man was a survivor, and nothing went to waste. I remember we had a large deep freezer that stored food in there since the Kennedy administration. They took me everywhere they went and they knew everyone in town. I learned so much from them; how to speak, how to read, to work, manners, and to love my family.

That kind of commitment carried on when my parents came for me and got married. They were ready to begin a new life with their little Macadoo (a nickname of mine...don't ask) outside the confines of Farmville. Five years later, my parents would give birth to Bit while we lived in Fort Hood, Texas, and again, in Aschaffenburg, Germany, to Jarvis five years later (my parents swear they didn't plan it that way).

In all that time, we had a wonderful childhood. And that is what I wanted for my child; the opportunity to give them the lessons I learned and the experiences I was exposed to; it made me who I am.

Now, that I am in my forties I am not sure if I am comfortable having a child. I can't speak for my wife, Sandra, who has written this book alongside me, I am sure with regret and heartache. For over the past 12 years we tried several times to conceive through natural means, three invitro fertility treatments, and three adoptions to no avail. Each attempt, no matter how we sought to have a child of our own was physically, financially, and emotionally trying. I felt like I was losing out on creating our own history.

I have never really had someone to talk to about our trouble with having children. I had no friends close enough to speak of it at the time, and I was not sure if my parents understood how Sandra would process that feeling of incompleteness. That feeling that she is less than a woman, and that somehow God was punishing her for some ill perceived transgression.

So we discussed it amongst ourselves, which I'm not sure if that was the right thing to do without seeking professional counsel first. So, we fought a lot. Not at first when we found out she could not have a child naturally, but when we began and failed through our first invitro attempt. If you don't know anything about the invitro fertilization process, keep reading my wife's perspective on the experience. It's a long arduous task of doctor visits, daily needles, and sometimes, uninspired hopes.

So many factors come into play on the creation of a child, not counting the financial toll which is immense and debilitating. I started to see cracks in her resolve; how useless she felt, and by extension how little or much (depending on her point of view at the time) I may have contributed to her pain. I wouldn't say we were blaming each other but there was definitely some resentment.

We didn't have much money at the time and our jobs weren't very helpful or sympathetic to our situation, which only caused more stress to our marriage. None was more devastating after our first attempt at invitro when Sandra lost the triplets a couple of months into the first trimester due to complications. To this day, well over 13 years ago, we still aren't sure what went wrong. Sandra and I were happy and proud that we were soon to become parents, but after the first month, Sandra started getting sick; to the point where she was unable to move her body without pain and was bedridden for the next two or three weeks. She couldn't sleep well, couldn't hold down food or water, and she was losing weight to the point of emaciation. I was scared; we both were. Our doctors kept telling us that everything was ok, when we saw clearly that something was wrong.

I was helpless to make anything right. I was in a new temp job that barely paid any money or provided adequate benefits for me let along another, and Sandra was running out of time to take off from work, otherwise, she might have lost her job. She was denied FMLA by the company; saying she did not qualify. What do you do? She can't go back to work in this condition! For whatever reason that I suspect had nothing to do with my performance but everything to do with their obligation to cover the cost of the procedure through my benefits, I lost my permanent job on the very day that my wife was implanted surgically with our fertile eggs to carry to term.

Now as a man, a husband, and a potential father I felt I was failing our future. It is no small thing when a man loses his ability to provide; especially when you have three new gifts arriving to sustain. But, sadly, none of that mattered. To our eventual heartbreak, we lost all three babies to some unknown complication.

After that, our home felt dark for a long time to which we have yet to recover fully. This terrible event has been the catalyst for our string of bad luck throughout our attempts to adopt or conceive a child through invitro for the last 12 years. Sandra was devastated by the loss, but I had to deal by being strong for her, and to convince her that this does not diminish her as a woman, all the while dealing with my own feelings of guilt and rage.

You start seeing friends of yours having children of their own and creating a culture that you do not feel a part of, but yearn for, despite your best efforts. Your family feels incomplete without a child, especially when it's not your choice. I cried some nights not long after; but it did not last long. I don't know why it does not stay with me like it used to but I didn't blame God or anyone else for our troubles. It is what it was supposed to be I believe. Maybe we weren't ready to bear children, but I still wanted to try. I was more concerned with Sandra's well-being and sanity than my own. Locked away and held in check until our crises abated... but not to disappear. It seems like a "man" thing to do, I know, but I had to be strong for the both of us in this situation. Some years later we have gotten better acclimated with one another with the fact that we would be without children in our lives, but there is still that lingering pain. It manifests itself with not necessarily just a feeling of acceptance of ones' fate, but the anxiety mortality.

The feeling that I will not be able to, in some way, raise a child to carry my name. I have no one to carry traditions and story of self to the rest of the world in a matter of speaking. My stem of the branch of our family tree ends with me. Sure my brothers have children of their own that will continue on as young men and women reaching for the sun. But my story ends as a fable that withers and falls when the seasons change never to re-emerge at the onset of spring; a supporting character of the main narrative that does not last long into the sequel, regardless of his importance.

My nieces and nephews will remember me of course but they carry the legacy of their parents to their children, not the uncle and aunt. It's a lonely existence that I am not sure I care to meet when I die. Then I ask myself, and this comes up from time to time between Sandra and I; should we try again in our declining prime years to bear children? I don't know. We have been through so much and I am not sure we can continue being disappointed.

It helps that we have Kali, our crazy cocker spaniel, that is as close to a child that we are ever going to have at this point, but she is a poor substitute for a child's first words, their first steps, or their first lie to you that they did not break the frame on your bed wrestling their cousins during a sleep over. Their joys and disappointments; the life worth lived as I have while growing up that when they are adults, they start sharing and laughing about all the ridiculous shit they did, and were supposed to do, while in your love and care. All that versus the life Sandra and I have now that we are able to leave on vacation when and wherever we want, to go out to a movie or dinner without looking for a babysitter, or not having to spend an incredible amount of money on medicine and childcare. Or, which is even scarier...raising them through adolescence.

I couldn't imagine growing up nowadays. It seems that there are more pedophiles, drugs, bullies, inept teachers and administrators, gang fights over the simplest of slights, and police shootings of young black men. It's more than I care to deal with, without my own share of violence to protect my child. And I know I won't be able to protect him or her from everything that comes along. Kids these days lack the one thing that my generation grew up on...constantly; a healthy dose of fear and respect. I can and will impart that upon my child; someone else's child, however, may not have that option, and worlds will collide. So the question remains, should we act in our own self-interest or should we chase immortality? It is the reason even Kings of old have sons to carry on their name and title to further their influence to the corners of their realm and beyond. How am I to deny that? It's almost inherent. It's why my father is proud of his children to this day; that when he passes from this plane of existence, he leaves a legacy of love and self that will impact generations of his significance.

I love my wife, I do. And I know the burden she carries of not providing...not immortalizing our lives for the next generation of Braxton's; so we find ourselves supporting, at scheduled times, caring for our nieces and nephews by taking them to Disneyland, cheering for them during their athletic games and activities, or gifts for their birthdays, and Christmas. I sometimes think she feels like Ellie from the animated movie, UP, from Disney and

Pixar. There is a scene during the beginning of the movie that resonates with Sandra and me, regarding the characters Ellie and Carl Fredricksen. If you have not watched this movie, please do so and you will see what I mean on how sad and unfair life can be to even the best of people. There is a happy ending, of course; hey, it's Disney. However, real life is never as pleasant as they portray it to be but, it makes a point.

Should the lack of having a child ruin who we are or how we spend our lives? I know my friends think we are living the good life but we are bereft of the experience of having a family and expanding our brand, as it were; but I am not sure if I want to deal with the complexities of raising a child at 50 or 60 years old. For now, I have dealt with my demons and have come to terms with having a limited family. I find solace in the knowledge that my brothers will carry on and raise their children, in some respects, as we were raised by our parents. And I am sure and gladdened by that fact that one day I can and will influence those kids with some nugget of myself that will serve them for the rest of their lives even when I have no child of my own to bear my soul to. Sandra and I will serve them for as long as we are able because we are a family.

ABOUT THE AUTHORS

Sandra M. Braxton is a Devoted wife and Entrepreneur based in Atlanta who owns a Travel Agency (The Braxton Agency) as well as a Jewelry boutique (Modest Trinkets). She is a Certified Project Manager with an MBA degree and is known for her outstanding organizational skills. Sandra is also an Air Force Gulf War Veteran that loves to give back to the Community. She participates yearly in the Strides for Breast Cancer walk, donates to UNCF, the Wounded Warrior campaign, March of Dimes, and so many others. Mentoring is one of her many passions. She recently joined ACP (American Corporate Partners) where she mentors Veterans transitioning into the Corporate world. Traveling the world brings her joy and so does spending quality time with like-minded individuals.

Octavian M. Braxton resides in Atlanta, with his wife, Sandra and their little beast of a dog, Kali, the Big Paw. He is a graduate of Mercer University, currently pursuing an advanced degree in Education and Liberal Studies, where he envisions a career as a professor with his Alma Mater. He is a Manager and mentor to kids and young adults whom he schools on life's educations and the decisions we make when faced with challenges against our destiny, however great or small. He is also a Veteran of the United States Air Force. He has travelled extensively throughout his life and wants to share his love of family and education with the next generation who sorely needs it.

You can get more information on the Braxton's Businesses by visiting their website www.thebraxtonconnection.com

CPSIA information can be obtained
at www.ICGtesting.com
Printed in the USA
LVHW080509240120
644690LV00012B/228

9 781518 742354